YOUR KNOWLEDGE HAS VALUE

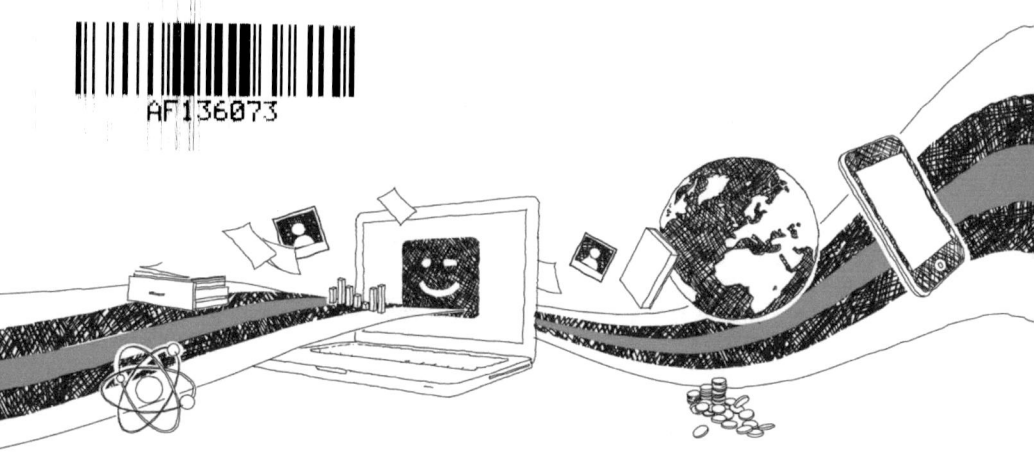
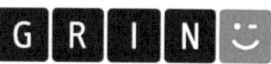

Assessment of the Epidemiological Approach in Surveillance of Notifiable Diseases in a Selected City in NCR (National Capital Region)

Basis For An Improved Disease Surveillance

Glen Samson

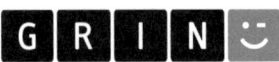

Bibliographic information published by the German National Library:

The German National Library lists this publication in the National Bibliography; detailed bibliographic data are available on the Internet at http://dnb.dnb.de.

ISBN: 9783346787590
This book is also available as an ebook.

© GRIN Publishing GmbH
Nymphenburger Straße 86
80636 München

Print and binding: Books on Demand GmbH, Norderstedt, Germany
Printed on acid-free paper from responsible sources.

The present work has been carefully prepared. Nevertheless, authors and publishers do not incur liability for the correctness of information, notes, links and advice as well as any printing errors.

GRIN web shop: https://www.grin.com/document/1308879

Assessment of the Epidemiological Approach in Surveillance of Notifiable Diseases in a Selected City in NCR: Basis For An Improved Disease Surveillance

Glen Dawi Samson, MPH, RMT, DTA

ABSTRACT

In the event of the ongoing pandemic, disease surveillance was one of the pillars in prevention of the spread of disease. The CoViD-19 pandemic was an eye opener for the whole world in which practice of disease surveillance was reevaluated for improvement. In the Philippines the disease surveillance encompasses the reporting of notifiable diseases which is important in controlling, preventing, and providing a response to the area that is affected by the disease that can possibly to result to death.

The objective of this study was to assess the epidemiological approach to surveillance of notifiable diseases in a selected city in NCR. There were one hundred ninety-six (196) respondents or 91% of the sample projection which were coming from different health facilities in the said City. This study emphasizes the importance of the Epidemiological approach in dealing with disease surveillance which will lead to disease containment and the establishment of an improved and strong epidemiological approach in assessing disease outbreaks. The result of the study will also help to promote the updating of protocols in disease surveillance and disease containment of notifiable diseases in cases of disease outbreaks, epidemics, and even pandemics. The study also provides the current assessment of the epidemiological approach in surveillance of notifiable diseases in a selected city in NCR in times of pandemic which will provide background for enhancement of the disease surveillance in line with the pandemic situation and infectious diseases that may arise anytime.

Keywords:

Epidemiological Approach, Notifiable Diseases, Disease Surveillance, Disease Outbreak, Surveillance System, Epidemiology, Pandemic, Epidemic, and Endemic

INTRODUCTION

Communicable diseases like the plague and bacterial infections dated back from classical times and are known even in the history of the bible. Cholera is also a bacterial infection from the 19th century that caused a million lives. Spanish flu is a viral disease caused by the H1N1 influenza virus that infected over 500 million people and over 100 million deaths from 1918 to 1920. Severe acute respiratory syndrome coronavirus (SARS-CoV) in 2002 and Middle East respiratory syndrome coronavirus (MERS-CoV) in 2012 were caused by a viral agent known as coronavirus that affects the respiratory tract, and now CoViD-19 in which many deaths have been recorded. These are well-known pandemics in the history of humanity and change the world in the perception of diseases (Sokol, 2020). A lot of human infectious diseases that lead to the pandemic are known to be caused by zoonotic pathogens that were transmitted to humans via close contact with animals (Piret & Bovin, 2021).

Disease outbreaks such as endemic, epidemic, and pandemic need to be addressed by a systematic approach that is well known for breaking the chain of infection in which case epidemiology is important. Epidemiology as part of public health that promotes disease investigation, prevention, control, and mitigation is essential in the provision of public health. In the Philippines, the International Health Regulations (IHR) of 2005 integrated a system that helps in the disease surveillance of notifiable diseases that is mandated to all WHO member states. This is to implement a set of international standards that has the goal of prevention, protection against the pathogen, controlling and providing public health response to the spread of disease. Disease surveillance is important for monitoring outbreaks and formulation of a time-efficient public health approach that will help in the prevention of the spread of the disease to the community. It also serves as a public health function in which it includes support for case detection and intervention, provides analysis of the impact of the disease, layout the distribution of cases, formulates hypotheses, stimulates prevention and control measures, and plans for further approaches.

Reporting notifiable diseases is important in controlling, preventing, and providing a response to the area that is affected by the disease that can result in death and even disease outbreaks. This can be achieved via a rapid recognition and timely reporting of information necessary for notifiable diseases (Nair & Ramdas, 2020). In addition to that, knowledge of the staff in charge of the surveillance of notifiable disease is vital to the timely reporting of the disease for the timeliness of the reporting is important in the disease surveillance and prevention of disease outbreaks in the affected area. Challenges and problems in disease surveillance of notifiable diseases are noted to be early detection, timeliness of reporting, ruling out a diagnosis, and long process of reporting that can affect the immediate response to the notifiable diseases (Do et al., 2020).

Furthermore, a commentary paper done by Buckee et al in 2018 emphasizes the problem of surveillance of notifiable diseases that are concerned with the process of reporting, the flow of the reporting, inadequacy of the data gathered, and the involvement of the government in the process of disease surveillance. Vital participation of every disease surveillance unit in the surveillance, monitoring, and containment of the disease is also noted in every part of the process. This relates to the situation of disease surveillance all over the world.

In the Philippines, a system for disease surveillance was established to help improve the response of the government to disease outbreaks and is known to be Philippine Integrated Disease Surveillance and Response (PIDSR). The data gathered by this system is being used for the public health decision-making of the government, for the detection and response to disease outbreaks. But the manual of Philippine Integrated Disease Surveillance and Response (PIDSR) is known to be inconsistent in its terms and description like the case of malaria in which it was categorized as category II as a weekly notifiable disease that uses Case Report Forms but malaria cases use Case Investigation Form that is used for Category I (Lopez et al., 2019). Despite this inconsistency, this system is still the one being utilized in the country as the primary tool in disease surveillance.

Inconsistent with the policy and approach in disease surveillance may lead to blind judgment of public health situations and may lead to disease outbreaks and even epidemics and pandemics. Training for this area of public health is also a vital part for the health workers so they will be able to identify and correctly diagnose the disease and do timely reports to respective departments to assist in immediate disease investigation and disease control that will lower the risk of a disease outbreak (Mairosi et al., 2017).

In the Republic Act, number 11332 known as "Mandatory Reporting of Notifiable Diseases and Health Events of Public Health Concern Act" reporting of notifiable diseases was emphasized, which mandates that all healthcare professionals and facilities accurately and immediately report a notifiable disease. That includes the 25 diseases enumerated in the Philippine Integrated Disease Surveillance and Response (PIDSR) manual of 2014 namely acute flaccid paralysis, adverse events following immunization (AEFI), anthrax, human avian influenza, measles, meningococcal disease, neonatal tetanus, paralytic shellfish poisoning, rabies, severe acute respiratory syndrome (SARS) are in the list categorized as immediate reporting is required in which case reporting of less than 24 hours is required in this category of disease. The other category in which weekly notifiable diseases namely acute bloody diarrhea, acute encephalitis syndrome, acute hemorrhagic fever syndrome, acute viral hepatitis, bacterial meningitis, cholera, dengue, diphtheria, influenza-like illness, leptospirosis, malaria, non-neonatal tetanus, pertussis, typhoid fever, and paratyphoid fever that are reported weekly. Furthermore, are these guidelines pertinent in the implementation of disease surveillance of notifiable diseases.

In addition, a report provided by Romulo Nieva in May of 2020 mentions one of the vital parts of disease prevention is a reliable system that can provide data rapidly and accurately which can provide immediate public health response. Disease containment, disease detection, and disease monitoring provide early identification of the disease outbreak. Policy and guidelines like the republic act number 11332 known as the "Mandatory Reporting of Notifiable Diseases and Health Events of Public Concern Act" which was passed last 2019 address the gaps in actions on disease outbreaks. Nevertheless, this is the real thing that is happening right now in the current situation of a pandemic.

In the study entitled early response to CoViD-19 in the Philippines by Amit, Pepito, and Dayrit in 2020, the authors mention various responses done by the government in the response to the pandemic like the travel restrictions and community quarantines that was imposed in the late phase of the pandemic. Lack of initial response to a public health threat like notifiable diseases can lead to community outbreaks and burden the community with the disease. Organizational preparedness like the detection of the disease and manpower in the provision of primary health care incapacitates the country to provide an immediate response to the pandemic.

This study emphasizes the importance of the Epidemiological approach in dealing with disease surveillance that will lead to disease containment and the establishment of an improved and strong epidemiological approach to assessing disease outbreaks. The result of the study will also help to promote the updating of the protocol in disease surveillance and disease containment of notifiable diseases in case of disease outbreaks, epidemics, and pandemics. The study also provides the current assessment of the epidemiological approach in surveillance of notifiable diseases in a selected city in NCR in times of pandemic which will provide background for enhancement of the disease surveillance in line with the pandemic situation and infectious diseases that may arise anytime.

Hypotheses of the Study

The researcher proposed the following hypotheses.

Ho1. There is no significant difference in the level of knowledge on disease surveillance when the respondents are grouped according to their profile.

Ho2. There is no significant difference in the level of satisfaction on the implementation of disease surveillance when the respondents are grouped according to their profile.

Ho3. There is no significant difference in the assessment of the effectiveness of the policies and guidelines in terms of epidemiological approach when the respondents are grouped according to their profile.

METHODOLOGY
Research Designs

The quantitative research method was utilized to obtain results that were logical, statistical, and unbiased for the assessment of the epidemiological approach to surveillance of notifiable diseases in a selected city in NCR.

Furthermore, the researcher utilized the Descriptive Evaluative and Comparative research design in the study commenced. Wherein, the descriptive evaluative research design was used to obtain data on the current nature and situation of the variable as the study was being conducted. This aims to describe what currently exists in the study variable (Lau & Kuziemsky, 2017). This descriptive evaluative design was utilized by the researcher in the study to describe the current assessment of the situation when it comes to disease surveillance in considering the level of knowledge of the respondents on disease surveillance, the implementation of policies in different health facilities in a selected city in NCR, and the disease surveillance system itself.

Moreover, the descriptive comparative design was utilized by the researcher to compare the data of different groups based on the parameters provided in the study (Lau & Kuziemsky, 2017).

The descriptive comparative design was used in the study to provide a comparison to the level of knowledge, policies, and system of disease surveillance in different health facilities to know what factors are different and what would be the implication of the difference in public health.

Locale of the Study

This study was conducted in one of the cities in NCR with 25 active health facilities for surveillance of notifiable diseases which encompasses the private and public health facilities with 215 personnel involved in disease surveillance. The purpose was to assess the Epidemiological approach to Surveillance of Notifiable Diseases in that chosen city.

The selected city in NCR is known for its immediate response to a public health concern, as the launching of online medical consultation as part of their city epidemiology and surveillance unit amid the initial spread of CoViD-19 in April 2020 to suppress the ongoing outbreak of the disease (Caliwan, 2020).

Furthermore, the establishment of the first Local Government Unit-owned molecular diagnostic laboratory that is situated within the city as part of their disease response was also noted for its public health concern.

The Population of the Study

The total number of respondents of the study were those who were involved in the disease surveillance from twenty-five (25) active health facilities for notifiable disease surveillance in one of the cities in NCR which has a total of 215 personnel involved in disease surveillance. In this sense, no sampling technique was used in the study for it used the total number of the population of the surveillance personnel in the locale of the study.

In addition to that, the list or number of personnel involved in the surveillance was provided by the facility to identify who were those person designated by them in the surveillance of notifiable disease as mandated by Republic Act 11332 and Philippine Integrated Disease Surveillance and Response (PIDSR) Manual of

Procedure in the establishment of the facility-based surveillance team.

In consideration of the respondents and administration to refuse to participate in the study, only 196 out of 215 answered the survey which is 91% of the total number of respondents as projected by the researcher.

Ethical Considerations

To secure the ethical integrity of the study it was subjected to compliance by the Institutional Ethics Review Committee of Our Lady of Fatima University and was approved. The researcher also secured informed consent form the respondents that their information was to be kept confidential. The following ethical principles are noted in the conduct of the actual study: autonomy, volunteerism, confidentiality, beneficence, non-maleficence, and originality.

Moreover, the survey tool used was validated by three (3) public health experts including a mental health coordinator that analyzed and checked if there was a mental health effect of the questions contained in the survey tool. In addition, briefing and debriefing of participants thru online video conference or phone calls regarding the study before and after participating in the study via the informed consent form in which contact details of the researcher for any inquiries regarding the study were provided. Furthermore, contact details of the Our Lady of Fatima University-Institutional Ethics Review Committee were also noted, accompanied by hotlines for mental health concerns.

This study was also subjected to a plagiarism or similarity test to secure the originality of the study in which the test yields an acceptable result of ten percent (10%) which was within the acceptable similarity index of Our Lady of Fatima University for Graduate School study of fifteen percent (15%).

Research Instrument

The survey tool was crafted by the researcher based on the Philippine Integrated

Disease Surveillance Response 2014 version with some additional data that was relevant to the disease outbreak at present. This research instrument was utilized to gather the required data from the respondents. The survey tool that was utilized had 4 different parts that helped in assessing the epidemiological approach to surveillance of notifiable diseases in a selected city in NCR.

Data Gathering Procedure

A letter of intent, request, and survey tool was handed out to the administrators or head of the health facility in a selected city in NCR that was active in disease surveillance to obtain an approval to proceed with the collection of data with the respondents in the health facility of concern. With permission of the facility administration, the survey tool and informed consent were sent to the respondents via a link or quick response (QR) code for the convenience of the respondents and for the health protocols to be observed during the implementation of community quarantine.

The link or quick response (QR) code was forwarded to the health facility focal person that led the respondents to the consent form and survey tool in google forms (https://docs.google.com/forms) an online survey platform that was accomplished online.

The data were gathered directly from the online platform in an excel format. It was further processed into a simplified and coded form to be utilized in the statistical analysis of the study. These data were also converted into numerical data and grouped according to the profile of the respondents to be used in the statistical analysis of the data for significant differences.

Data Analysis

The results and findings of the study were subjected to organizing and tabulation to be used in the statistical analysis in which computation and interpretation of raw data were done with appropriate tools.

Frequency counts and the percentage were to describe the profile of the respondents. While weighted mean and standard deviation were utilized to describe the assessment of the respondents of their level of knowledge on disease surveillance, implementation of disease surveillance, and effectiveness of the policies and guidelines in terms of the epidemiological approach that provide primary data that was utilized further with another statistical tool.

To calculate the level of knowledge of the respondents to the disease surveillance in terms of the following variables namely: notifiable diseases; disease prevention and control, disease containment; disease detection; disease reporting; timeliness of reporting; and epidemiology. This measures the level of knowledge by a scale determined by the Likert system which was utilized to provide a range wherein the weighted mean of the areas was interpreted as to the values of the Likert scale as seen in the scale below.

Knowledge Scale

Scale	Level of knowledge	Value
4	Very Knowledgeable	3.26 – 4.0
3	Knowledgeable	2.52 – 3.25
2	Minimal Knowledge	1.76 – 2.51
1	Not Knowledgeable	1.0 – 1.75

The implementation of disease surveillance which was furthermore subdivided in terms of organizing the surveillance system, cooperation and coordination surveillance system, process of surveillance, epidemiology and surveillance training, monitoring and evaluation of the surveillance system, and manner of reporting. These were measured with four (4) levels which are delineated as "very satisfactory" as the highest parameter designated as 4, followed by "satisfactory" designated as 3, followed by "unsatisfactory" designated as 2, and last and least was "very unsatisfactory" designated as 1. These values were assessed in the study as to the scale below with the use of the Likert system.

Satisfaction Scale

Scale	Level of Satisfaction	Value
4	Very satisfactory	3.26 – 4.0
3	Satisfactory	2.52 – 3.25
2	Unsatisfactory	1.76 – 2.51
1	Very unsatisfactory	1.0 – 1.75

In the assessment of disease surveillance personnel as to the policies and guidelines in the epidemiological approach in surveillance of notifiable diseases in the selected city in NCR. These were measured with four (4) levels which are delineated as "very effective" as the highest parameter designated as 4, followed by "effective" designated as 3, followed by "ineffective" designated as 2, and last and least was "very ineffective" designated as 1. These values were assessed in the study as to the scale below with the use of the Likert system.

Effectiveness Scale

Scale	Level of Effectiveness	Value
4	Very Effective	3.26 – 4.0
3	Effective	2.52 – 3.25
2	Ineffective	1.76 – 2.51
1	Very Ineffective	1.0 – 1.75

One Way Analysis of Variance (ANOVA) was used to determine if there was a significant difference in the level of knowledge of disease surveillance, implementation of disease surveillance, and effectiveness of the policies and guidelines in terms of epidemiological approach when grouped according to their profile.

The Scheffe test was utilized as a post hoc test to look for the groups that have significant differences after the one-way analysis of variance (One-way ANOVA) which provided primary data that the groups had a significant difference. This test was best utilized with data that were not normally distributed across groups and all possible simple and complex groups were analyzed. A T-test was also utilized to determine the significant difference between the two groups denoting the health facility classification.

One Way Analysis of Variance (ANOVA), Scheffe test, and T-test provided the ruling in which acceptance or rejection of the hypothesis will depend on.

RESULTS

Demographic Profile

The succeeding was the summary finding of the study correspondingly based on the demographic profile of the respondents. With regards to professions wherein, *Barangay Health Workers (BHW)* logged the highest response and the least were *Medical Technologists*. As to the age bracket, the majority of the respondents were from *51 to 55 years old* and least from *20 to 25 years old* and *36 to 40 years old*. In the matter of training and seminars relevant to disease surveillance or infection control for the past 3 years, the highest frequency was from those who *do not have training at all* and the least was from those who were *with training for the past 3 years*. In reference to the years of service as part of the surveillance team, the most logged response was from those who were in the team for about *0 to 5 years* and the least was from *16 to 20 years.* and in connection with health facility classification wherein the majority of the respondents came from the *public health facility* while a smaller portion came from the *private health facility*.

Level of Knowledge of The Respondents on Disease Surveillance

Based on the results of the study the respondents' assessment when it comes to their knowledge of disease surveillance in terms of notifiable disease (WM=2.90), disease prevention and control (WM=2.91), disease containment (WM=2.86), disease detection (WM=2.83), disease reporting (WM=2.86), timeliness of reporting (WM=2.96), and epidemiology (WM=2.87) that yield most answers that were knowledgeable with regards to these parameters of disease surveillance. In addition, an overall weighted mean of 2.87 was yielded in this parameter that showed that the disease surveillance personnel in the selected city in NCR was knowledgeable when it comes to disease surveillance of notifiable diseases using the Likert system to interpret the data provided.

Level of Satisfaction of the Respondents on the Implementation of Disease Surveillance

As for the result of the study wherein satisfaction with the implementation of the disease surveillance in the selected city in NCR was considered, it revealed that the disease surveillance personnel were satisfied with the implementation of the disease surveillance that yielding an overall weighted mean of 2.86 which was satisfactorily using the Likert system. Furthermore, each parameter organizing the surveillance system (WM= 2.9), cooperation and coordination surveillance system (WM= 2.92), the process of surveillance (WM= 3.01), epidemiology and surveillance training (WM= 2.73), monitoring and evaluation of the surveillance system (WM= 2.83), and manner of reporting (WM= 2.75) which also yield individual assessment of satisfactory using the Likert system.

Assessment of the Respondents on the Effectiveness of Policies and Guidelines in Epidemiological Approach in Surveillance of Notifiable Diseases

With regards to the outcome of the study, it showed that the respondents of the study, mainly the disease surveillance personnel answered that the policies and guidelines in the epidemiological approach to surveillance of notifiable diseases were effective with a weighted mean of 3.04 was equivalent to effective using the Likert system.

Significant Difference in the Level of Knowledge of The Respondents on the Disease Surveillance

Upon consideration of the demographic profile of the respondents, there was a significant difference seen in the level of knowledge of the disease surveillance personnel using the ANOVA with an additional statistical test of Scheffe test to locate where the significant difference lies when it comes to profession, training, and seminars relevant to disease surveillance, and years in service as part of the surveillance team. The

significant difference in the profession wherein barangay health workers have a significant difference with dentists (Scheffe value = 87.18), medical technologists (Scheffe value = 82.52), midwives (Scheffe value = 127.86), nurses (Scheffe value = 32.83) and physician (Scheffe value = 82.52). There was also a significant difference with nursing aides to midwives (Scheffe value = 22.30) and physicians (Scheffe value = 59.44). Another was also revealed with a nurse and physician (Scheffe value = 46.55).

Moreover, the significant difference seen in the level of knowledge of disease surveillance personnel when training and seminars relevant to disease surveillance were considered was seen with those who doesn't have training at all and those who doesn't have for the last three (3) years (Scheffe value = 80.90) and those who had their seminar and training within the span of three (3) years (Scheffe value = 220.59). An additional significant difference was also noted between those who do not have for the last three (3) years and those who had their seminar and training within the span of three (3) years (Scheffe value = 31.58).

In addition to that, the significant difference recorded when the years of service as part of the surveillance team of the disease surveillance personnel was considered revealed that 0-5 years of service as part of the surveillance team has a significant difference with those who were in the service for 11-15 years (Scheffe value = 59.50), 16-20 years (Scheffe value = 154.94), 21 years and above (Scheffe value = 66.70). Another significant difference was seen between those who were in the service for 6-10 years and 16-20 years (Scheffe value = 24.28).

Meanwhile, in the level of knowledge of the respondents to the disease surveillance the age group in the demographic profile of the disease surveillance personnel does not have a significant difference when put into consideration using the ANOVA. And there was no significant difference in the level of knowledge of the respondents about the disease surveillance when the health facility classification was considered with the use of the T-test.

Significant Difference in the Level of Satisfaction of The Respondents on the Implementation of Disease Surveillance

What's more, regards to the satisfaction of the respondents with the implementation of the disease surveillance in the selected city in NCR was a significant difference when the demographic profile of the respondents was considered. The ANOVA revealed that there was a significant difference when profession, age, and training and seminars relevant to disease surveillance were considered and these groups were further subject to Scheffe test wherein it showed which groups had a significant difference.

As for the profession the significant difference lies between barangay health worker and dentists (Scheffe value = 59.03), medical technologists (Scheffe value = 66.14), midwives (Scheffe value = 18.44), nurses (Scheffe value = 25.30), nursing aides (Scheffe value = 14.70) and physician (Scheffe value = 52.16). As for the age group, 56-60 years old has a significant difference with 46-50 years old (Scheffe value = 19.83), 51-55 years old (Scheffe value = 27.09), and 61 years old and above (Scheffe value = 29.77). As for the training and seminar relevant to disease surveillance significant difference was seen with those who does not have training at all and those who does not have for the last three (3) years (Scheffe value = 10.82) and those who had their seminar and training within the span of three (3) years (Scheffe value = 101.54). The additional significant difference was also noted between those who did not have for the last three (3) years and those who had their seminar and training within the span of three (3) years (Scheffe value = 42.40).

Apart from the mentioned above, there was no significant difference in the satisfaction with the implementation of disease surveillance when years in service as part of the surveillance team were analyzed using ANOVA and health facility classification analyzed using T-test in consideration with the demographic profile of the respondents.

Significant Difference in the Assessment of the Respondents on the Effectiveness of the Policies and Guidelines in Terms of Epidemiological Approach

Along with this assessment of effectiveness, a further analysis using ANOVA was utilized in this area to check if there was a significant difference when the demographic profile of the respondents was considered. The analysis using ANOVA revealed a significant difference when profession, age, and training and seminars relevant to disease surveillance were noted.

In considering the profession, a significant difference was seen between barangay health workers and dentists (Scheffe value = 14.82), medical technologists (Scheffe value = 41.95), midwives (Scheffe value = 34.73), nurses (Scheffe value = 20.60), and physician (Scheffe value = 31.37). With regards to the age group, ages 56-60 years old has a significant difference with 61 years old and above (Scheffe value = 24.42). And for the training and seminar relevant to disease surveillance significant difference was seen between those who does not have training at all and those who does not have for the last three (3) years (Scheffe value = 30.22) and those who had their seminar and training within the span of three (3) years (Scheffe value = 30.22).

Aside from the data above, there was no significant difference in the assessment of the effectiveness of the policies and guidelines in the epidemiological approach in surveillance of notifiable diseases seen in the years in service as part of the surveillance team when subjected to ANOVA and health facility classification when subjected to T-test with regards to the consideration of the disease surveillance personnel demographic profile.

DISCUSSION

The objective of this study was to assess the epidemiological approach to surveillance of notifiable diseases in a selected city in NCR. There were one hundred ninety-six (196) respondents or 91% coming from different health facilities. The analysis tools used to treat the data were frequency, percentage, weighted mean, standard deviation, One Way ANOVA, and T-test. The results showed that barangay health workers (27%) dominated with the highest number of respondents. Most of the disease surveillance personnel were from the 51-55 years of age (22%); for the respondents training and seminars relevant to the disease surveillance and infection control for the last three (3) years, most of them did not have any training or seminar at all (45%). With regards to the years in service as part of the surveillance, the majority of the respondents answered 0-5 years (60%) for they can be considered newbies as disease surveillance personnel. And for the health facility classification, more than half of the respondents came from the public health facility (63%).

On top of that, the disease surveillance personnel in the selected city in NCR were knowledgeable when it comes to the basics of the disease surveillance mainly with notifiable diseases (WM=2.90; SD=0.97), disease prevention and control (WM=2.91; SD=0.91), disease containment (WM=2.86; SD=0.92), disease detection (WM=2.83; SD=0.91), disease reporting (WM=2.86; SD=0.92), timeliness of reporting (WM=2.96; SD=0.96), and epidemiology (WM=2.75; SD=0.93) that resulted of an overall weighted mean of 2.87 with standard deviation of 0.93.

This study also revealed that the level of satisfaction of the respondents in the implementation of disease surveillance in one of the cities in NCR in terms of the organization of the surveillance system (WM=2.9; SD=0.74), cooperation and coordination surveillance system (WM=2.92; SD=0.74), the process of surveillance (WM=3.01; SD=0.73), epidemiology and surveillance training (WM=2.73; SD=0.75), monitoring and evaluation of the surveillance system (WM=2.83; SD=0.81), and manner of reporting (WM=2.75; SD=0.81) was all satisfactory with an overall weighted mean of 2.86 and standard deviation of 0.77. While the assessment of the respondents on the policies and guidelines in the epidemiological approach to surveillance of notifiable diseases was assessed as effective, with a weighted mean of 3.04 and standard deviation of 0.71.

Significant differences were also noted with these parameters about their groups based on their demographic profile. The significant difference in the level of knowledge of the respondents to the disease surveillance was noted with regards to their profession (p value=0.00), training and seminars relevant (p value=0.00), and years in service as part of the surveillance team (p value=0.00). In the part of the level of satisfaction on the implementation of disease surveillance in which significant differences in the demographic profile of the respondents like the profession (p value=0.00), age (p value=0.00), and in the training and seminars relevant to the disease surveillance (p value=0.00) was shown in the study. Meanwhile, the part of the assessment of policies and guidelines in which significant differences were revealed in the demographic profile of the respondents for the profession (p value=0.00), age (p value=0.00), and in the training and seminars relevant to disease surveillance (p value=0.00).

This study can be encapsulated that the respondents were knowledgeable enough about the parameters of the disease surveillance given in this study. The respondents of the study were also satisfied with the implementation of the disease surveillance in their facility and local area. And the respondents also considered that the policies and guidelines in line with the epidemiological approach in the surveillance of notifiable diseases were effective in their facility and the local area as the time of the study was conducted.

CONCLUSION

In the demographic profile wherein the profession of the disease, surveillance personnel were dominated by barangay health workers with the highest number of recorded responses. As for the age groups considered, most of the disease surveillance personnel were from 51-55 years of age which was most of the responses submitted. When it comes to the training & seminars relevant to disease surveillance, and infection control for the last 3 years, most of the respondents do not have any training or seminar at all. With regards to the years in service as part of the surveillance team, the major bulk of the respondents answered 0-5 years for they can be considered newbies as disease surveillance personnel. And for the health facility classification, wherein more than half of the respondents came from the public health facility.

The disease surveillance personnel in the local area of the study were knowledgeable when it comes to the fundamentals of the disease surveillance mainly with notifiable diseases, disease prevention and control, disease containment, disease detection, disease reporting, timeliness of reporting, and epidemiology. For major bulk of the responses from the respondents that they are knowledgeable with regards to these parameters of disease surveillance.

The assessment of the level of satisfaction of the respondents on the implementation of disease surveillance in the local area of the study was revealed as satisfactory, especially with regards to organizing the surveillance system, cooperation and coordination surveillance system, process of surveillance, epidemiology and surveillance training, monitoring and evaluation of the surveillance system, and manner of reporting. These were reflected in the majority of the response of the disease surveillance personnel with the parameters noted above.

This study also revealed that the disease surveillance personnel in the local area of the study assessed the policies and guidelines in the epidemiological approach in surveillance of notifiable diseases as effective in their facility and the local area.

In the level of knowledge of the disease surveillance personnel, there was a significant difference in their profession, training, and seminars relevant to disease surveillance, and years in service as part of the surveillance team.

As to the level of satisfaction with the implementation of the disease surveillance in the local area of the study, there was a significant difference in the profession, age, and training and seminars relevant to disease surveillance.

The study also revealed a significant difference in the profession, age, and training and seminars relevant to disease surveillance in the assessment of the effectiveness of the policies and guidelines in terms of epidemiological approach.

Above all, the study conducted presented results that can be put into a nutshell the disease surveillance personnel of the local of the study were knowledgeable about the parameters given in the study the disease surveillance and were also satisfied with the implementation of the disease surveillance in their facility and in their local area, and lastly that the policies and guidelines in line with the epidemiological approach in the surveillance of notifiable diseases were effective as of the time that the study was conducted.

RECOMMENDATIONS

In view of the study, the researcher would like to suggest the following recommendations to provide a better epidemiological approach to surveillance of notifiable diseases:

1. Provision of training and seminars to the disease surveillance personnel were huge aid in the detection, prevention, and mitigation of notifiable disease in a certain area.

2. Combination of paper-based and electronic-based reports can generate a good quality record of the information for it also serves as a back-up for the record.

3. Guidelines and policies for disease surveillance should be up to date and parallel to the ongoing situation of diseases that are emerging and re-emerging.

4. Strengthen the implementation of the disease surveillance system via health promotion, disease

prevention, control in the area, and education with regards to the notifiable diseases for the betterment of the locality that can be patterned by the other city and even in the national government to provide aid in the establishment and updating of the system in their respective areas.

5. An aging number of disease surveillance personnel should be addressed by recruiting and training new personnel to take over the task in the near future.

6. Promote general information with regards to the relevance of disease surveillance to the health of every individual in the community.

7. Encourage the Master in Public Health professionals and students to engage in the prevention and control of diseases via disease surveillance to aid the possible workforce drain due to the age of the disease surveillance personnel.

8. Stimulate the general public and non-health facilities to engage in disease surveillance for a better and more effective disease surveillance system in the locality they belong to.

9. And lastly, the researcher would like to encourage future researchers to conduct a qualitative study to know further information with regards to the data reflected in this study. It is also recommended for them to take part in expanding the knowledge in improving disease surveillance not only in the country but up to the international level.

Authors' Contributions:

Dr. AGNES A. GUZMAN, his adviser for all the prompting, aid, perseverance, diligence, and a pillar in executing this study.

The Faculty, Chair and the Members of the Panel from the Graduate School of Our Lady of Fatima University, for contributing their critique, knowledge, and expertise to enhance and improve the study.

REFERENCES:

Abdulrahim, N., Alasasfeh, I., Khader, Y. S., & Iblan, I. (2019). Knowledge, awareness, and compliance of disease surveillance and notification among jordanian physicians in residency programs. INQUIRY: The Journal of Health Care Organization, Provision, and Financing, 56, 004695801985650. https://doi.org/10.1177/0046958019856508

Abrigo, M. R. M., & Ortiz, D. A. P. (2019). Philippine Institute for Development Studies DISCUSSION PAPER SERIES NO. 2019–32. Who Are the Health Workers and Where Are They? Revealed Preferences in Location Decision among Health Care Professionals in the Philippines, DISCUSSION PAPER SERIES NO. 2019–32, 10–13. https://pidswebs.pids.gov.ph/CDN/PUBLICATIONS/pidsdps1932.pdf

Ahmed, N., Shakoor, M., Vohra, F., Abduljabbar, T., Mariam, Q., & Abdul Rehman, M. (2020). Knowledge, awareness and practice of health care professionals amid SARS-CoV-2, corona virus disease outbreak. Pakistan Journal of Medical Sciences, 36(COVID19-S4). https://doi.org/10.12669/pjms.36.covid19-s4.2704

Amit, A. M., Pepito, V. C., & Dayrit, M. (2021). Early response to COVID-19 in the Philippines. Western Pacific Surveillance and Response Journal, 12(1), 56–60. https://doi.org/10.5365/wpsar.2020.11.1.014

Arada, M. A. B., & Jose, S. M. L. (2020). Assessment of the knowledge, attitude and practice of pregnant women towards hepatitis b infection seen at a tertiary hospital in the Philippines. Published. http://www.pjog.org/download.php?id=215

Bagherian, H., Farahbaksh, M., Rabiei, R., Moghaddasi, H., & Asadi, F. (2017). National communicable disease surveillance system: a review on information and organizational structures in developed countries. Acta Informatica Medica, 25(4), 271. https://doi.org/10.5455/aim.2017.25.271-276

Caliwan, C. L. (2020, April 6). Marikina launches online medical consultation amid Covid-19. Philippine News Agency. https://www.pna.gov.ph/articles/1098949

Centers for Disease Control and Prevention. (2013). Overview of evaluating Surveillance systems. Www.Cdc.Gov. Retrieved April 25, 2022, from https://www.cdc.gov/globalhealth/healthprotection/fetp/training_modules/12/eval-surv-sys_fieldg_final_09262013.pdf

Collado, Z. C. (2019). Challenges in public health facilities and services: Evidence from a geographically isolated and disadvantaged area in the philippines. Journal of Global Health Reports, 3. https://doi.org/10.29392/joghr.3.e2019059

de Guzman, C. (2018, June). Embracing new healthcare technologies that empower Filipinos. PwC Philippines. https://www.pwc.com/ph/en/pwc-needles-in-a-haystack/embracing-new-healthcare-technologies-that-empower-Filipinos.html

Do, H., Ho, H. T., Tran, P. D., Nguyen, D. B., Otsu, S., de Vázquez, C. C., Dang, T. Q., Tran, Q. T., Pham, V.

A., Mikami, N., & Kato, M. (2020). Building the hospital event-based surveillance system in Viet Nam: a qualitative study to identify potential facilitators and barriers for event reporting. Western Pacific Surveillance and Response Journal, 11(3), 10–20. https://doi.org/10.5365/wpsar.2019.10.1.009

Dodd, W., Kipp, A., Nicholson, B., Lau, L. L., Little, M., Walley, J., & Wei, X. (2021). Governance of community health worker programs in a decentralized health system: a qualitative study in the Philippines. BMC Health Services Research, 21(1). https://doi.org/10.1186/s12913-021-06452-x

Douglas, T. A., Pooley, J. A., Shields, L., Stick, S. M., & Branch-Smith, C. (2021). Early disease surveillance in young children with cystic fibrosis: A qualitative analysis of parent experiences. Journal of Cystic Fibrosis, 20(3), 511–515. https://doi.org/10.1016/j.jcf.2020.10.001

Ducomble, T., & Gignoux, E. (2020). Learning from a massive epidemic: measles in DRC. The Lancet Infectious Diseases, 20(5), 542. https://doi.org/10.1016/s1473-3099(20)30265-6

El Allaki, F., Bigras-Poulin, M., Michel, P., & Ravel, A. (2012). A population health surveillance theory. Epidemiology and health, 34, e2012007. https://doi.org/10.4178/epih/e2012007, Retrieved August 14, 2021, https://www.ncbi.nlm.nih.gov/pmc/articles/PMC35 21104/

Garg, S., Bhatnagar, N., & Gangadharan, N. (2020). A case for participatory disease surveillance of the covid-19 pandemic in India. JMIR Public Health and Surveillance, 6(2), e18795. https://doi.org/10.2196/18795

Grayson, M. L., Stewardson, A. J., Russo, P. L., Ryan, K. E., Olsen, K. L., Havers, S. M., Greig, S., & Cruickshank, M. (2018). Effects of the australian national hand hygiene initiative after 8 years on infection control practices, health-care worker education, and clinical outcomes: a longitudinal study. The Lancet Infectious Diseases, 18(11), 1269–1277. https://doi.org/10.1016/s1473-3099(18)30491-2

Groseclose, S. L., & Buckeridge, D. L. (2017). Public Health Surveillance Systems: Recent Advances in Their Use and Evaluation. Annual Review of Public Health, 38(1), 57–79. https://doi.org/10.1146/annurev-publhealth-031816-044348

Hardhantyo, M., Djasri, H., Nursetyo, A. A., Yulianti, A., Adipradipta, B. R., Hawley, W., Mika, J., Praptiningsih, C. Y., Mangiri, A., Prasetyowati, E. B., & Brye, L. (2022). Quality of National Disease Surveillance Reporting before and during COVID-19: A Mixed-Method Study in Indonesia. International Journal of Environmental Research and Public Health, 19(5), 2728. https://doi.org/10.3390/ijerph19052728

Haw, N. J. L., Uy, J., Sy, K. T. L., & Abrigo, M. R. M. (2020). Epidemiological profile and transmission dynamics of COVID-19 in the Philippines. Epidemiology and Infection, 148. https://doi.org/10.1017/s0950268820002137

Ibrahim, L. M., Stephen, M., Okudo, I., Kitgakka, S. M., Mamadu, I. N., Njai, I. F., Oladele, S., Garba, S., Ojo, O., Ihekweazu, C., Lasuba, C. L. P., Yahaya, A. A., Nsubuga, P., & Alemu, W. (2020). A rapid assessment of the implementation of integrated disease surveillance and response system in Northeast Nigeria, 2017. BMC Public Health, 20(1). https://doi.org/10.1186/s12889-020-08707-4

Ilmakunnas, P., & Ilmakunnas, S. (2018). Health and retirement age: Comparison of expectations and actual retirement. Scandinavian Journal of Public Health, 46(19_suppl), 18–31. https://doi.org/10.1177/1403494817748295

Jiang, L., & Huang, T. (2019). Comparison of the epidemiological aspects of acute infectious diseases between foreign and native imported cases in the border counties of Southwest China, 2008–2017. Epidemiology and Infection, 147. https://doi.org/10.1017/s0950268819001195

Jinadu, K. A., Adebiyi, A. O., Sekoni, O. O., & Bamgboye, E. A. (2018). Integrated disease surveillance and response strategy for epidemic prone diseases at the primary health care (PHC) level in Oyo State, Nigeria: what do health care workers know and feel? Pan African Medical Journal, 31. https://doi.org/10.11604/pamj.2018.31.19.15828

Karimuribo, E. D., Mutagahywa, E., Sindato, C., Mboera, L., Mwabukusi, M., Kariuki Njenga, M., Teesdale, S., Olsen, J., & Rweyemamu, M. (2017). A smartphone app (afyadata) for innovative one health disease surveillance from community to national levels in Africa: intervention in disease surveillance. JMIR Public Health and Surveillance, 3(4), e94. https://doi.org/10.2196/publichealth.7373

Khan, H., Khan, S., & Iqbal, A. (2009). Knowledge, attitudes and practices around health research: the perspective of physicians-in-training in Pakistan. BMC Medical Education, 9(1). https://doi.org/10.1186/1472-6920-9-46

Ladner, J. T., Grubaugh, N. D., Pybus, O. G., & Andersen, K. G. (2019). Precision epidemiology for infectious disease control. Nature Medicine, 25(2), 206–211. https://doi.org/10.1038/s41591-019-0345-2

Lau F, Kuziemsky C, editors. Handbook of eHealth Evaluation: An Evidence-based Approach [Internet]. Victoria (BC): University of Victoria; 2017 Feb 27. Available from: https://www.ncbi.nlm.nih.gov/books/NBK481590/

Lin, C., Braund, W. E., Auerbach, J., Chou, J. H., Teng, J. H., Tu, P., & Mullen, J. (2020). Policy Decisions and Use of Information Technology to Fight Coronavirus Disease, Taiwan. Emerging Infectious Diseases, 26(7), 1506–1512. https://doi.org/10.3201/eid2607.200574

Long, C., Liu, P., & Yi, C. (2020). Does educational attainment affect residents' health? Healthcare, 8(4), 364. https://doi.org/10.3390/healthcare8040364

Madhav, N., Oppenheim, B., Gallivan, M., Mulembakani, P., Rubin, E., & Wolfe, N. (2017). pandemics: risks, impacts, and mitigation. disease control priorities, third edition (volume 9): improving health and reducing poverty, 315–345. https://doi.org/10.1596/978-1-4648-0527-1_ch17

Mallari, E., Lasco, G., Sayman, D. J., Amit, A. M. L., Balabanova, D., McKee, M., Mendoza, J., Palileo-Villanueva, L., Renedo, A., Seguin, M., & Palafox, B. (2020). Connecting communities to primary care: a qualitative study on the roles, motivations and lived experiences of community health workers in the Philippines. BMC Health Services Research, 20(1). https://doi.org/10.1186/s12913-020-05699-0

McIntosh, T. (2020). The impact of technological advances on older workers. Walden Dissertations and Doctoral Studies Collection. https://scholarworks.waldenu.edu/cgi/viewcontent.cgi?article=10679&context=dissertations

Moise-Silverman, J. (2022). Zoonotic disease surveillance and response: Is there a duty to intervene when a disease is detected? International Journal of Infectious Diseases, 116, S77. https://doi.org/10.1016/j.ijid.2021.12.182

Murray, J., & Cohen, A. L. (2017). Infectious disease surveillance. international encyclopedia of public health, 222–229. https://doi.org/10.1016/b978-0-12-803678-5.00517-8

Mwabukusi, M., Karimuribo, E. D., Rweyemamu, M. M., & Beda, E. (2014). Mobile technologies for disease surveillance in humans and animals. Onderstepoort J Vet Res, 81(2). https://doi.org/10.4102/ojvr.v81i2.737

Nair, S., & Ramdas, I. (2020). Profile of communicable diseases reported under integrated disease surveillance programme in a teaching hospital. Journal of Family Medicine and Primary Care, 9(8), 4165. https://doi.org/10.4103/jfmpc.jfmpc_552_20

Nieva, R. F. (2020, May). Robust disease surveillance and 'outbreak drill'. The Philippine News Agency. https://www.pna.gov.ph/opinion/pieces/296-robust-disease-surveillance-and-outbreak-drill

Nilsson, E., & Nilsson, K. (2017). The transfer of knowledge between younger and older employees in the health and medical care: An intervention study. Open Journal of Social Sciences, 05(07), 71–96. https://doi.org/10.4236/jss.2017.57006

Nnebue, C., Onwasigwe, C., Onyeonoro, U., & Adogu, P. U. (2012). Awareness and knowledge of disease surveillance and notification by health-care workers and availability of facility records in Anambra state, Nigeria. Nigerian Medical Journal, 53(4), 220. https://doi.org/10.4103/0300-1652.107557

Ogugua, I., Chime, O., Obionu, I., Ezenwosu, I., Ibiok, C., Ochie, C., Kassy, W., Ndu, A., Arinze-Onyia, S., Agwu-Umahi, O., Aguwa, E., & Okeke, A. (2021). Assessment of knowledge and practice of disease surveillance and notification among health workers in private hospitals in Enugu State, Nigeria. Nigerian Journal of Medicine, 30(6), 693. https://doi.org/10.4103/njm.njm_132_21

Phalkey, R. K., Yamamoto, S., Awate, P., & Marx, M. (2013). Challenges with the implementation of an Integrated Disease Surveillance and Response (IDSR) system: systematic review of the lessons learned. Health Policy and Planning, 30(1), 131–143. https://doi.org/10.1093/heapol/czt097

Piret, J., & Boivin, G. (2021). Pandemics throughout history. frontiers in microbiology, 11. https://doi.org/10.3389/fmicb.2020.631736

Querri, A., Ohkado, A., Kawatsu, L., Bermejo, J., Vianzon, A., Recidoro, M. J., & Medina, A. (2020). Assessment of the role of community health volunteers in delivering primary health care in Manila, the Philippines. Journal of International Health, 35(1), 15–25. https://doi.org/10.11197/jaih.35.15

Raghupathi, V., & Raghupathi, W. (2020). The influence of education on health: an empirical assessment of OECD countries for the period 1995–2015. Archives of Public Health, 78(1). https://doi.org/10.1186/s13690-020-00402-5

Razu, S. R., Yasmin, T., Arif, T. B., Islam, M. S., Islam, S. M. S., Gesesew, H. A., & Ward, P. (2021). Challenges faced by healthcare professionals during the COVID-19 pandemic: A qualitative inquiry from Bangladesh. Frontiers in Public Health, 9. https://doi.org/10.3389/fpubh.2021.647315

Richards, C. L., Iademarco, M. F., Atkinson, D., Pinner, R. W., Yoon, P., Mac Kenzie, W. R., Lee, B., Qualters, J. R., & Frieden, T. R. (2017). Advances in Public Health Surveillance and Information Dissemination at the Centers for Disease Control and Prevention. Public Health Reports, 132(4), 403–410. https://doi.org/10.1177/0033354917709542

Salvador, Roderick; Tanquilut, Neil; Lampang, Kannika Na; Chaisowwong, Warangkhana; Pfeiffer, Dirk; and Punyapornwithaya, Veerasak, "Identification of high-risk areas for the spread of highly pathogenic avian influenza in Central Luzon, Philippines" (2021). Journal Article. 243. https://www.ukdr.uplb.edu.ph/journal-articles/243

Sayono, S., Widoyono, W., Sumanto, D., & Rokhani, R. (2019). Impact of Dengue Surveillance Workers on Community Participation and Satisfaction of Dengue Virus Control Measures in Semarang Municipality, Indonesia: A Policy Breakthrough in Public Health Action. Osong Public Health and Research Perspectives, 10(6), 376–384. https://doi.org/10.24171/j.phrp.2019.10.6.08

Senate and House of Representatives of the Philippine Congress Assembled. (2019, April 26). Republic act No. 11332 "Mandatory Reporting of Notifiable Diseases and Health Events of Public Health Concern Act." The LawPhil Project Arellano Law Foundation. Retrieved August 20, 2021, from https://lawphil.net/statutes/repacts/ra2019/ra_11332_2019.html

Society for Community Health Awareness Research and Action. (n.d.). How to organise epidemiological surveillance system. Https://Www.Sochara.Org/Clic_pubblication/Edu_materials/218. Retrieved April 25, 2022, from http://sochara.org/uploads/aboutuploads/AyddRa_7.%20How%20to%20organise%20an%20epidemiological%20surveillance%20system.pdf

Taburnal, M. V. M. (2020). Knowledge and competence of barangay health workers (BHWS). International Journal of Innovation, Creativity and Change, 14(1), 1301–1320. https://www.ijicc.net/images/Vol_14/Iss_1/14160_Taburnal_2020_E_R.pdf

Tayag, E. et al, (2014). Manual of procedures for Philippine integrated disease surveillance and response

(PIDSR) 3rd Edition April 2014 National
Epidemiology Center, Department of Health,
Philippines retrieved from
https://doh.gov.ph/node/9985

The Lancet Infectious Diseases. (2019). Infectious disease
crisis in the Philippines. The Lancet Infectious
Diseases, 19(12), 1265.
https://doi.org/10.1016/s1473-3099(19)30642-5

Toda, M., Zurovac, D., Njeru, I., Kareko, D., Mwau, M., &
Morita, K. (2018). Health worker knowledge of
Integrated Disease Surveillance and Response
standard case definitions: a cross-sectional survey at
rural health facilities in Kenya. BMC Public Health,
18(1). https://doi.org/10.1186/s12889-018-5028-2

Turner, S., Segura, C., & Niño, N. (2021). Implementing
COVID-19 surveillance through inter-
organizational coordination: a qualitative study of
three cities in Colombia. Health Policy and
Planning, 37(2), 232–242.
https://doi.org/10.1093/heapol/czab145

Vera EV, Monzon RB. An assessment of barangay health
midwives' knowledge regarding tuberculosis case
finding and treatment procedures in urban health
centers of metropolitan Manila, Philippines.
Southeast Asian J Trop Med Public Health. 1995
Dec;26(4):648-54. PMID: 9139369.

Vraukó, K., Jancsó, Z., Kalabay, L., Lukács, A., Maráczi, G.,
Mester, L., Nánási, A., Rinfel, J., Sárosi, T., Tamás,
F., Varga, A., Vitrai, J., & Rurik, I. (2018). An
appraisal: how notifiable infectious diseases are
reported by Hungarian family physicians. BMC
Infectious Diseases, 18(1).
https://doi.org/10.1186/s12879-018-2948-5

World Health Organization. (2016). International Health
Regulations (2005) (3rd ed.). World Health
Organization.

Youssef, D., Khoury, C., Allouch, G., Haydar, K., Jouny, A.,
Zreik, H., Ghoussaini, F., & Yaghi, A. (2018). Use
of District Health Information System (DHIS-2) for
Real Time Surveillance: Lebanon 2017.
Iproceedings, 4(1), e10547.
https://doi.org/10.2196/10547

Appendix: Survey Questionnaire

Please answer the questions by putting a check (√) about Demographic profile according to your knowledge. If you need clarification, please do not hesitate to ask the principal investigator.
PART I Demographic Profile
Demographic Profile – Respondents

1.1. Profession
( ) Physician   ( ) Nurse   ( ) Medical Technologist   ( ) Midwife   ( ) Radiologic Technologist
            ( ) Nutritionist & Dietician   ( ) Nursing Aide   ( ) Physical Therapist ( ) Others (Please indicate): _____

1.2. Age
( ) 20-25 yrs. old   ( ) 26-30 yrs. old   ( ) 31-35 yrs. old   ( ) 36-40 yrs. old   ( ) 41-45 yrs. Old
( ) 46-50 yrs. old   ( ) 51-55 yrs. old   ( ) 56-60 yrs. old   ( ) 61 yrs. old and Above

1.3. Trainings & seminars relevant to the disease surveillance, infection control for the last 3 years
( ) No training at all   ( ) None for the past 3 years   ( ) With Training & Seminar for the past 3 years

1.4. Years in service as part of the surveillance team
( ) 0-5 years   ( ) 6-10 years   ( ) 11-15 years   ( ) 16-20 years   ( ) 21 years and above

1.5. Health Facility Classification
( ) Private   ( ) Public

PART II. Knowledge on Disease Surveillance
This part of the survey will assess the knowledge of the respondents to disease surveillance. Kindly put a check on the box (√) that you see fit in your situation.
4 = Know about it   3 = Know little about it   2 = I have heard about it   1= No idea about it

Do you know or have background of the following?	4	3	2	1
2.1. Notifiable Diseases				
2.1.1. List of notifiable Diseases				
2.1.2. Categories of Notifiable Diseases				
2.1.3. Mode of Transmission of Notifiable Diseases				
2.1.4. Case Definition of Notifiable Diseases				
2.1.5. Tests to be done in a Notifiable Disease				
2.2. Disease Prevention & Control				
2.2.1. Minimum Health Standard or Protocol to be done in case of notifiable diseases				
2.2.2. Non-Pharmaceutical Interventions				
2.2.3. Possible Sources of infection				
2.2.4. Proper Reporting of a Case				
2.2.5. Who to Contact in Case of notifiable Disease				
2.3. Disease Containment				
2.3.1. Proper Containment of infected Individuals				
2.3.2 Time Frame of Infection				
2.3.3. Who to Consider as Close Contact				
2.3.4. Proper Decontamination and Sanitation of Area of Infection				
2.3.5. Preparations for a Notifiable Disease Event				
2.4. Disease Detection				
2.4.1. Proper Identification of the Disease				
2.4.2. Signs and Symptoms to Look for				
2.4.3. Specimens to be Collected				
2.4.4. Radius of Disease Surveillance in a Notifiable Disease Event				

2.4.5. Availability of the test for notifiable disease				
2.5. Disease Reporting				
2.5.1. Case Investigation Forms to be filled out				
2.5.2. Case Report Forms to be Filled out				
2.5.3. Event-Based Surveillance Report				
2.5.4. Flow of Reporting				
2.5.5. Agencies to Report to				
2.6. Timeliness of Reporting				
2.6.1. Reporting of category 1 of notifiable diseases (acute flaccid paralysis, adverse events following immunization (aefi), anthrax, human avian influenza, measles, meningococcal disease, neonatal tetanus, paralytic shellfish poisoning, rabies, severe acute respiratory syndrome (SARS)) **within 24 hours to the local epidemiology**				
2.6.2. Reporting of category 2 of notifiable diseases (acute bloody diarrhea, acute encephalitis syndrome, acute hemorrhagic fever syndrome, acute viral hepatitis, bacterial meningitis, cholera, dengue, diphtheria, influenza like illness, leptospirosis, malaria, non-neonatal tetanus, pertussis, typhoid fever, and paratyphoid fever) **within a week of the infection to the local epidemiology**				
2.6.3. In the event of flooding or typhoon leptospirosis and dengue and malaria are reported **within 24 hours**				
2.6.4. Reporting to the national level limits within 24 to 48 hours in the event of category 1 notifiable diseases.				
2.6.5. Weekly reporting of zero (0) cases with category 1 and 2				
2.7. Epidemiology				
2.7.1. Public Health Surveillance				
2.7.2. Collection of Epidemiological Data				
2.7.3. Disease Monitoring				
2.7.4. Analysis and Evaluation of Epidemiologic Data				
2.7.5. Public Health Interventions				

PART III. Implementation of Disease Surveillance
This part of the survey will assess the respondent's implementation of disease surveillance in the facility where he/she belong and the local area that the facility belongs to. Kindly put a check on the box (√) that you see fit in your situation
4 = Very satisfactory   3 = Satisfactory   2 = Unsatisfactory   1= Very unsatisfactory

Implementation of Disease Surveillance	4	3	2	1
3.1 Organizing the Surveillance System				
3.1.1. Organizational Structure of Surveillance System in your Facility				
3.1.2. Organizational Structure of Surveillance System in your Local Area				
3.1.3. Number of Personnel in your Structure of Surveillance System in Your Facility				
3.1.4. Number of Personnel in your Structure of Surveillance System in Your Local Area				
3.1.5. Coordination committees and meetings of surveillance system in your Facility and in your local area				
3.2 Cooperation and Coordination Surveillance System				
3.2.1. Cooperation and coordination in disease surveillance in your facility				
3.2.12 Cooperation and coordination in disease surveillance in your Local Area				
3.2.3. Confidence and participation of health staffs in your facility				
3.2.4. Confidence and participation of health staffs in your Local Area				
3.2.5 Flow of reporting in your facility and in your local area				
3.3 The Process of Surveillance				
3.3.1. Process of Identification of Notifiable Disease in your Facility				
3.3.2. Proper Documentation of the health event				
3.3.3. Reporting of Health event in your facility				
3.3.4. Reporting of Health event in your area				

3.3.5. Method of reporting in your facility and in your local area				
3.4 Epidemiology and Surveillance Training				
3.4.1. Assess your knowledge and training on epidemiology and disease surveillance				
3.4.2. Provision of Training or Seminar relevant to Epidemiology by your facility				
3.4.3. Provision of Training or Seminar relevant to Epidemiology by your local Area				
3.4.4. Provision of Training or seminar relevant to Disease Surveillance by your facility				
3.4.5. Provision of Training or seminar relevant to Disease Surveillance in your local area				
3.5 Monitoring and evaluation of the surveillance system				
3.5.1. Your facility Monitors and evaluate the surveillance system that is being implemented in the facility				
3.5.2. Your local area Monitors and evaluate the surveillance system that is being implemented in the facility				
3.5.3. Your local area Conduct regular technical assistance visits of your facility with the epidemiologist				
3.5.4. Your facility checks for the completeness of the disease investigation and reports				
3.5.5. Your local Area checks for the completeness of the disease investigation and reports				
3.6 Manner of Reporting				
3.6.1. Utilization of Written Paper-Based Report within the Facility				
3.6.2. Utilization of Online Electronic-Based Report within the Facility				
3.6.3. Utilization of Written Paper-Based Report within the Local Area				
3.6.4. Utilization of Online Electronic-Based Report within the Local Area				
3.6.5. Reporting Flow and Process within the Local Area				

PART IV. POLICIES AND GUIDELINES

This part of the survey will assess the effectiveness of the policies and guidelines that are being implemented in terms of epidemiological approach. Kindly put a check on the box (√) that you see fit in your situation

4 = Very Effective   3 = Effective   2 = Ineffective   1= Very Ineffective

Policies and Guidelines	4	3	2	1
Policies and Guidelines in epidemiological approach in surveillance of notifiable diseases (RA 11332 (Mandatory Reporting of Notifiable Diseases and Health Events of Public Health Concern Act), diseases surveillance, and investigation, testing of a notifiable disease, monitoring of notifiable diseases, and reporting of notifiable diseases.)				

I certify the answers to the above questions are correct to the best of my knowledge and any questions left unanswered may be discussed in any interview arising from this questionnaire.

Signed: _____   *Date:* _____